How to Red[...]
Sugar Cr[...]

Stop That Sugar Habit Controlling Your Life
and Break Your Sugar Addiction Forever

2

Table of Contents

Introduction

Sugar is an ingredient that causes much controversy today. We are used to consuming it, and it is in almost all of our food, whether we know it or not. Many people today treat all the food we eat differently, and ask questions about the consumption of sugar.

The consumption of sugar is related to causing both obesity and diabetes, two of the biggest problems of modern man. Is sugar really more dangerous than alcohol and tobacco? Is it an addiction? How can you get rid of this addiction?

Are these questions justified at all? From personal experience, I can tell you that they are.

In all my life, I have never been too fat. We can say that, as far as the weight goes, everything looked normal. With a height of 5'11" and weight of 209 lbs., I was not too bothered. Yet as the years passed, I realized that I'm not exactly in the best physical shape. What was happening too was that just a small climb up the stairs to the second floor, and I already could not catch my breath. It made me feel a little guilty, I am still young, but I moved around like an old man.

Then, I came somewhat to my senses, and started paying a little more attention to myself and to my body. I began to actively train, go to the gym, and to swim. I avoided fast-food restaurants, and I improved my diet a little, but this did not help much.

I did end up with a little better physical condition, but my weight still remained unchanged. I did not know exactly what was I doing wrong. Then, on a website, I accidentally saw that it all could have happened because of an excessive intake of sugar.

Then I stopped eating sweets and candy of any kind, but I felt desperate. I felt a constant need to eat or drink something sweet. Sometimes, the desire was so strong that I even felt physically ill. In such situations, I allowed myself to eat something sweet, but it would only be enough for a short time, and the cycle repeated. I simply couldn't find a way out.

Then my friends started saying that it was simply because of those few extra pounds that I had, and they recommend some of the popular diets. I opted for one of the popular protein diets.

At first, it seemed like it really worked. I began to lose weight, I had less desire for sugar, and for a moment, I even felt better. But this was for a very short time. This was quickly followed by severe headaches and fatigue. I soon did not even have the strength to get out of bed.

When the doctor examined me and looked at my blood tests, he almost tumbled out of his chair. My whole body was in complete chaos. I instantly stopped dieting, and everything returned to my old ways. I kept spinning in this unhealthy cycle.

People have suggested that I should use a variety of artificial sweeteners instead of sugar, but that did not seem healthy either.

Then I decided to take the matter into my own hands all the way. I began to investigate and to consult with various doctors and specialists in the field in order to find a method that would enable me to live a healthy life.

I'll be telling you all about the conclusions I came to during this process, and I'll point you to the methods I used to reduce and eliminate my sugar cravings. Also, I'll explain the mistakes that I made along the way, so you will not repeat them.

Chapter 1: What Is Sugar Exactly?

200 years ago, the average man would eat two pounds of sugar per year. In 1970, this amount was increased to 120 pounds per year. Today, the average person annually consumes more than 165 pounds of pure sugar!

In nature, there are simple and complex sugars. The most common simple sugars (monosaccharide) are glucose, fructose, and galactose. The complex sugars (disaccharides) are sucrose (ordinary table sugar), lactose (milk sugar), and maltose. Although we usually refer only to white sugar as sugar, all of these are actually forms of sugar.

Glucose is found naturally in plants, fruits, and vegetables, resulting from the process of photosynthesis. Our body burns glucose to obtain energy, or it stores it in the form of glycogen (fuel for the muscles and liver). When necessary, our body can mobilize glucose by breaking down the reserves of glycogen.

Fructose is fruit sugar. This means that you can find it there in all the fruits, but also in sugar cane, honey, and high fructose corn syrup (HFCS). It is sweeter than regular sugar.

Sucrose is ordinary table sugar (otherwise, raw sugar is 99.5% pure sucrose). Structurally, it consists of one molecule of glucose and fructose, linked by chemical bond. This chemical bond is broken into acidic solutions during chewing, digestion, and the like. Dr. Robert Lustig says that it takes about two seconds for sucrose to dissolve into glucose and fructose.

Lactose is milk sugar. It is less sweet than sucrose. It consists of one molecule of galactose and glucose linked by a chemical bond. For breaking this bond, the enzyme lactase is required. In babies and children, this enzyme is increased, while with age, the body decreases the secretion of lactase (lactose intolerance).

What Happens When You Eat Sugar?

When you eat sugar, glucose very quickly finds its way into the bloodstream. At that moment, the pancreas secretes the insulin hormone, which is responsible for removing glucose from the blood and changing it into a form which will later be used for energy. The more sugar you eat, the more glucose will be in your blood and, consequently, more insulin is released.

At this time, the sugar that is inside your body can use for energy or convert it to a fatty acid and store it in the form of body fat. The problem is that we often take in more sugar than the body needs at that moment. When there is too much sugar, insulin release is increased, which leads to the rapid removal of glucose from the blood, with the result that the sugar in blood drops below normal levels. When blood sugar is below the normal level, we feel like there is a fall in our energy (also known as low sugar). The result is that we eat sugar again, and everything repeats in a cycle. It is this dependence on sugar that everyone is talking about.

The more often this circuit is repeated, the more your body gets accustomed to the excess sugar not being used for energy, but immediately being stored as body fat.

Glycemic Index

That's not even the whole story. Our body also produces sugar from other food that we eat. Food from which our body produces only sugar is rich in complex carbohydrates - starches, potatoes, bread, pasta, and flour.

Surely you've heard of the glycemic index of food. The glycemic index is the indicator which shows us at what speed food rich in carbohydrates turns into sugar. If the glycemic index (GI) of food is higher, it means that it will more quickly be converted to sugar. Mashed potatoes and white bread have almost the same GI as pure sugar. Therefore, for example, it is better to eat whole meal bread (which has a lower GI than white bread), because it contains vegetable fibers that slow down the process of converting starch to sugar - and when the sugar is released slowly, your body has a constant, but not excessive flow of energy (when it is too large, and not used in the form of physical activity, for example, then this energy is converted to fat).

Of course, this does not mean that you should never again eat potatoes or pasta. I believe that carbohydrates should not be thrown out completely from your diet, but you should eat those carbohydrates that give you a steady stream of energy. Glycemic Load is a measure that determines the speed at which a meal is converted into sugar. If, along with pasta (foods with a high GI), you eat vegetables (with a low GI), it will have the cumulative effect of some middle GI. Also, for example, fruit juice has a higher GI than pure fruit - because the fruits have specific fibers that slow down the absorption of sugar into the blood.

Why Do We Eat Sweets After a Meal?

Typically for a meal, if you eat food rich in readily available carbohydrates (mashed potatoes, pasta, white bread), soon after that you might feel a need to eat something sweet (because insulin has already removed most of the sugar from the blood). Also, and this might seem somewhat paradoxical, if the meal was too big, you will also experience an urge for something sweet (too much food also leads to an increased secretion of insulin). So, add some fresh vegetables and protein on your plate, do not eat like this is your last meal in life, and there is no physiological reason that you would feel any kind of craving for something sweet after a meal.

If, after a moderate, balanced meal you still want to eat something sweet, experts in the field of nutrition agree -

it's a habit. It's a habit we have acquired from childhood to eat something sweet after a meal. Now that you know that it is a habit, not a physiological need, it will be somewhat easier to stop the habit.

Chapter 2: How Dangerous Is Sugar?

Sugar is dangerous if you consume it a lot. As with all things, if you do not overdo it, it is not dangerous. The FDA recommends that the amount of added sugar should not be higher than six tablespoons a day for women and nine for men. That much is packed into one can of Coke or a chocolate bar. But the more you eat the more, you get used to it, and the vicious cycle repeats. Although many stories about sugar are rather inflated, like the one that it causes hyperactivity in children (It does not cause hyperactivity, it is only a current influx of energy. Basically a hyperactive child now has more energy to be hyperactive), the fact is that today we do consume too much sugar.

How Exactly Does Diabetes Occur?

Given that we are saying that sugar, as we use it today, can cause diabetes, I think that it is very important that we know what this condition is. I think that the knowledge of this disease and the awareness that more and more people are struggling with is the final factor that has startled me from my "sugary dream." If you are still unsure whether I was right when it comes to the sugar we eat, allow me to describe how diabetes generally occurs.

When glucose, through a process of digestion, gets into the blood, it is transported to the cells where energy is needed. For glucose molecules to enter the cell in which they will break and release energy, insulin is necessary. Insulin is a hormone secreted by the pancreas. Insulin is secreted the moment that the level of glucose in the blood increases. If the blood does not excrete enough insulin, or it cannot for some reason achieve its effect, the cells that need energy are not able to take glucose molecules from the blood, and thus the level of glucose in the blood is constantly elevated above the normal range. This condition is called diabetes.

Because insulin cannot then help cells to utilize glucose, the whole body begins to feel weakness and fatigue. Then the cells send a signal that they need extra energy, and extra amounts of glucose gets into the blood, but due to insufficient levels of insulin (or lack of response to its effects) cells are still unable to take glucose from the blood. The organism perceives the increased amount of glucose in the blood as a risk, and with a large amount of liquid, it starts to remove glucose from the blood through the urine. Hence, one of the symptoms of diabetes is increased thirst due to dehydration. Other symptoms of diabetes include increased urination, fatigue, and weight loss.

All of this can lead to serious problems and consequences if not treated properly. People can become blind due to diabetes, or have their legs amputated. Not all people get diabetes because of the desire for sweets, but it is certain that such a type of sugar does not help, but increases our propensity for developing the disease.

Chapter 3: How to Stop the Addiction

The addiction to sugar is stopped by simply slowly "forgetting" the taste of sugar over time. Eat more vegetables, nuts, and dairy products (for example, whey protein increases the production of serotonin - a hormone that is released when we eat something sweet, and which induces the feeling of happiness). Whenever you think you have a sugar crash and that you need to eat something sweet, eat a handful of almonds, drink tea, lemonade, or yogurt.

As noted above, this dependence is not so much an addiction as it is a habit. They say that it takes three weeks to acquire new habits. During the course of three weeks remove sugar from your house (if you do not have candy at home, the idea is that you won't go to pick them up or you will burn some calories while doing so). For these three weeks, you will teach yourself primarily (and your own body) that you don't need sugar at the level which you have previously consumed.

Why Do You Feel Good When You Eat Something Sweet?

As we said before, simple carbohydrates start a series of chemical processes in our bodies that ultimately leads to raising the level of serotonin in our brain. Studies show that low levels of serotonin are among the main causes of cravings for sweets. Serotonin is a neurotransmitter that creates a sense of peace and contentment. The more serotonin you have, the happier you will feel. It is that simple.

Therefore, when we need a rapid growth of serotonin, we seek food that is rich in sugar. Unfortunately, the most sugar is found in processed food with lots of calories and few nutrients.

Excessive consumption of food containing simple carbohydrates can cause many health problems. Among them are diabetes, obesity, and heart disease.

And not only that - it was found that consumption of white sugar inhibits our ability of immunity so that we cannot fight infections, it can cause liver damage, disrupt the hormonal system, and increase the risk of cancer. If we concede too much to our craving for sugar in processed foods, we will cause a fast growth, followed by the equally rapid drop in blood glucose. This sharp drop, as mentioned before, encourages an even greater need for sugar, so it creates a vicious circle.

Just by eating healthy food that prevents sugar cravings and with enough exercise you can break this circle, as many nutritionists say. I myself found this to be true through my own fight with sugar.

Complex carbohydrates or polysaccharides, produce the same effect in terms of serotonin, they just do it slowly. I know that we live in a fast world, but a little patience can make this life healthier, and quite long.

Basic Steps for Quitting Sugar

These are some of the basic steps for quitting sugar, which I also applied. Do not take them as strict rules. These are more like the guidelines and principles that you have to apply in your life to be able to live healthy and free of sugar.

Do not skip meals

Eat three big meals and two small snacks a day, or five small meals a day. If you do not eat on time, there will be a fall in the level of sugar, and then comes the hunger and the greater likelihood that a craving for sweets will appear.

Choose unprocessed food

The more your food is close to its natural form, the more it will contain less refined sugar. Natural food does not present any metabolic problem for our body, especially if you eat a variety of different types and if you eat moderately.

Eat protein, fat, and phytonutrients for breakfast

A typical breakfast full of carbohydrates and sugar or starch is the worst possible choice to start the day - after that you will long for sugar all day. A good breakfast will prevent this desire.

Try to include protein and / or fat with each meal

This will help in controlling blood sugar levels. Be careful to only eat healthy fats like avocado or olive oil and healthy forms of protein.

Add spices

Coriander, cinnamon, nutmeg, and cardamom will naturally sweeten food and reduce cravings for sugar.

Check whether you are suffering from a lack of vitamins or minerals

If you miss some nutrients, the craving for sugar can be increased. Certain substances such as vitamin B3 and magnesium help to maintain a stable blood sugar level.

Move around

Use any form of exercise or movement that you love to reduce tension, increase energy, and reduce the need for sugar.

Get enough sleep

Sleep-deprived people are more likely to eat sugar to suppress the feeling of fatigue.

Do not buy candy

Do not keep in your home any sweets and sugary cereals. It's hard to nibble on something that is not there.

Do not use artificial sweeteners

Besides not being the healthiest, artificial sweeteners do not reduce the craving for sugar, they just mask it. If you must, use stevia, it is the healthiest substitute sugar.

Read labels

It is best to eat less food that has labels, but when you are buying food at least read the composition. The longer the list of ingredients, the more likely that the list has sugar in some form. Do not buy foods in which sugar is listed in the first three ingredients. Choose the ones with the least amount of sugar.

Identify the names behind which sugar also hides

These are some of the ingredients that are basically sugar: corn syrup, corn sugar, sucrose, dextrose, honey, molasses, turbinado sugar, and brown sugar.

Disguised sugar

Most of the "complex" carbohydrates that we eat such as bread, biscuits, and pasta are not complex. They are usually highly refined and in our body, they act like sugar. They should be avoided. It is also important to know what to do if you do get a craving for sugar.

Short break

Find a quiet and comfortable place. Sit down a minute, and concentrate on your breathing. The craving will pass in a few minutes.

Change your thoughts

Take a walk, if possible in nature, and if you're in the city, take the streets which do not have any kind of food vendor. Cravings can take a maximum of 10 to 20 minutes. Have some fun, and your craving will probably pass.

Drink lots of water

Sometimes drinking water helps, because sometimes, while we feel the desire to eat, we are actually being thirsty.

Eat a piece of fruit

If you cannot resist the desire, at least eat the healthiest form of sugar - fruit.

If you follow this advice, you may occasionally give up and treat yourself to ice cream. Do not feel bad, ice cream is nice and fun, just make sure that you balance it out during the day.

Chapter 4: A Healthy Substitute for Sugar

The following foods will satisfy your cravings without harm to your health.

Tomatoes

Tomatoes are effective against cravings for sugar, because they contain high levels of tryptophan - substances that the body converts into serotonin. This fruit (yes a tomato is a fruit - get over it) is rich in chromium, a mineral that reduces the craving for food and regulates cholesterol and blood glucose levels.

Apples

One of the best fruits to satisfy the desire for sweets is the apple. It's easy to carry and does not need to be peeled or cut as other fruits. Even the sour varieties of apples contain a lot of healthy carbohydrates. This fruit is rich in dietary fibers, which gives a feeling of satiety and reduces hunger.

Sweetcorn

Sweet corn is yet another healthy food that can help in the "withdrawal from sugar." It abounds in antioxidants, vitamins, minerals, and dietary fiber. In addition to the urge to eat sugar, it also reduces hunger.

Sweet Potatoes

Another vegetable that can help is sweet potatoes. This food will not only satisfy your craving for sugar, but will additionally provide the body with vitamin C, D, B6, and iron. Nutrients in sweet potatoes can prevent heart disease, cancer, and other degenerative diseases.

Cinnamon

Cinnamon is a fantastic spice that has an excellent flavor and aroma, so you can add it to many dishes. Cinnamon helps against a great desire for sugar. This spice prevents sudden fluctuations in blood glucose levels that contribute to sugar cravings, thus delaying the need for injecting a new portion of sugar. Cinnamon helps the efficiency of insulin, thereby helping the organism to convert glucose into energy. Cinnamon simultaneously helps to prevent coronary artery disease, and high blood pressure. Cinnamon can be sprinkled over cereal, fruit, yogurt, or toast ... Strive to eat a quarter of a teaspoon of cinnamon daily.

Fish

Fish in the diet can prevent the development of type 2 diabetes. Researchers concluded that people who regularly eat fish have 50% less likelihood to develop diabetes than those who do not eat it at all. Omega 3 fats from fish can stimulate the body's ability to use glucose, and thus prevent the onset of diabetes. The amount which has a protective effect is very small, and is only one ounce a day of sea fish, but without the addition of other fats other than olive oil.

Dandelion

The ingredient that may sound strange to you is Dandelion. In addition to being a useful natural remedy for liver and gall bladder, this herb is a good natural remedy for controlling blood sugar levels. For the treatment of diabetes, it is necessary, during the spring, to eat 10 fresh dandelions every day. You should previously wash the whole plant with its flower and only then remove the flowers. Then slowly chew and swallow the rest of the plant.

These foods will not only reduce the craving for sweets, but will also improve your health and maintain a slim waistline.

As an alternative to white sugar, when preparing cakes and desserts, you can use maple or agave syrup, stevia, and coconut sugar.

Chapter 5: Correlation Between Food Cravings and Lack of Nutrients

Most people have a need or desire for a particular food, even when they are not hungry. The good news is that in most cases the craving for food is derived from the simple physiological or psychological causes, and can be controlled by introducing the necessary nutrients to the body.

It is very important to have healthy food at hand in times of crisis to be a great substitute for the unhealthy ones which are usually our first choice.

Salty Snacks

The need for chips, popcorn, f and other salty snacks indicates certain shortcomings related to the adrenal gland and the lack of electrolytes. It often occurs because of a hormonal imbalance due to stressful situations. An increased need for salt intake usually indicates the body's need for electrolytes and minerals. The craving for salt may also mean that the body cries for water, since salt tends to encourage water retention.

Increase fluid intake. Consume celery, olives, tomatoes, seaweed, or Himalayan salt to compensate electrolytes and minerals. Ensure enough sleep and rest for your body, which will normalize levels of stress hormones in the body.

Carbohydrates: Bread, Pasta, Biscuits

Your thoughts are preoccupied with pasta, cakes, breads, crackers and rolls? This may be an indicator of insulin resistance, hypoglycemia (sudden drop in blood sugar levels), chromium deficiency, or chronic fatigue. Most likely, you need an additional intake of chromium and balance sugar levels in the body. Eat bananas, apples, apricots, spinach, beets, avocados, broccoli, celery, chard, carrots, and parsnips. To better control the sugar in your diet, include more fiber. To overcome the craving for carbohydrates, eat more dark green vegetables, and foods rich in chromium and magnesium. Ensure your intake of small amounts of protein with every meal (soy, legumes, or dairy products).

Chocolate

If you crave for chocolate, it is likely that your body lacks magnesium, essential fatty acids, and chromium. In times of stress, the body has lowered levels of magnesium, chromium, B vitamins, and essential fatty acids. That is why we, when we get exposed to stress, reach for chocolate to make up for a lack of these nutrients.

But that's not all - chocolate increases serotonin levels in the blood. Since serotonin is the hormone of happiness, craving for chocolate may be associated with emotional needs.

Consume hot chocolate made from raw cocoa, nuts and seeds, legumes, green leafy vegetables, and other foods rich in magnesium and essential fatty acids.

A great solution is talking with loved ones and friends, or engaging in any activity that will raise serotonin levels and contribute to a good mood.

Sweets

You cannot live a day without sweets? This means that your body needs extra energy, chromium, or an essential amino acid tryptophan. Craving for sweets is perhaps one of the most complex nutritional needs. It may indicate a lack of amino acids or fungal growth in the body. Also, a greater need for sweets or sugar can be a sign that your body needs carbohydrates as energy for the brain and body. The desire for sweet foods can be an emotional character that lacks the "sweetness" in your life. Consume beans, pears, berries, pumpkin seeds, sunflower seeds, and whole grains.

Treat yourself to activities that will cheer you up and relax, such as a walk in nature, art, or good music, and you will notice that the craving for sweets can be satisfied without food.

Fried and Fatty Foods

Longing for fried and fatty food indicates a lack of essential fatty acids, or a calcium deficiency. Eat nuts and seeds, flax oil, broccoli, kale, legumes, and green leafy vegetables.

Carbonated Drinks

The craving for soft drinks is often present in people who take too many stimulants in their body, and at the same time do not drink enough water. This could be a sign of a lack of calcium in the body. Consume kale, almonds, spinach, and broccoli which will help replace calcium.

Ice

Craving for ice, clay, earth, chalk, and other non-food products is a condition that is also called Pica or Geophagia (which literally means "eat dirt"). It can often indicate a lack of iron or other minerals in the body. This phenomenon is more common in children, but can occur in adults during periods of increased nutritional needs, such as pregnancy. Eat more iron-rich foods, including dark green leafy vegetables, legumes, nuts, and seeds.

When you experience cravings for food, do not ignore them or simply comply. Listen to what your body tells you, and find the best way to give it what it desires. This is one of the major conclusions it has reached by itself. We're used to everything being at our disposal, and we respond to every situation by satisfying our needs without thinking.

Chapter 6: A Couple of Useful Recipes

When I got into the whole process of research about the withdrawal of sugar and a healthy diet, a friend who is a professional chef gave me a couple of recipes that have helped me to combine healthy foods and clean my body of sugar. He dealt with a lot of traditional cuisine of various world nations and has pulled food and meals out of their folklore that have served this purpose, sometimes for centuries back.

I will share several of those recipes with you now.

Soup for Lowering Blood Sugar

Necessary ingredients:

- 2 cups of water

- 1 unpeeled onion cut into four parts

- 17.6 ounces of beans

- 1 small carrot cut into cubes

- 1/2 cup of peanuts

- 1/2 cup of sprouts of fenugreek or 1/2 teaspoon of fenugreek seed

- 2 bay leaves

- 4 cloves of chopped garlic

- A pinch of ground cinnamon

- A pinch of ground cloves

- A pinch of turmeric.

Preparation:

In a large saucepan, over medium heat, cook the onion in the water until it boils. Add beans, carrots, peanuts, sprouts, or seeds of fenugreek, bay leaf, garlic, cinnamon, cloves and turmeric. When it boils, cook over low heat for 30 minutes or until the onion becomes quite soft. Remove the pieces of onion, peel and throw the shell. Lightly mash the onion with a fork and return it to the saucepan. Remove the bay leaf and throw them away.

The amount of soup is enough for 4 people.

Horseradish, Garlic and Beer

Necessary ingredients:

• Horseradish root length of about 7.8 inches and a thickness of about 0.78 inches.

• 9 cloves of garlic.

• Fresh quality beer.

• Glass 32-ounce jar or bottle.

Thoroughly wash, but do not peel the horseradish roots. Finely chop it, and place it in the jar. Peel and wash the cloves of garlic. Chop them up and put them in the jar. Pour the fresh beer (up to the narrowing of the jar), cover with something and leave in a dark place for 10 days. Strain afterwards.

Intake:

The first 2 days: 1 teaspoon, 2-3 times a day,

The next few days: per 1 tablespoon, 3 times a day before meals.

This mixture can "lower" high blood sugar within a month and keep it under control.

Porridge for Reducing Blood Sugar Levels

• Pour 1.7 ounces of oat grains with 16 ounces of boiled and cooled water.

• Put on the quiet fire, bring to a boil and cook for 10-15 minutes.

• Remove from heat, cover and leave it for 1 hour

Take half a glass 3-4 times a day before meals.

The duration of the treatment: 2-3 weeks.

Super Eggs

Whisk 1 egg. Squeeze juice from 1 medium lemon into the egg.

Thoroughly mix the ingredients.

Take: every morning on an empty stomach. Duration of treatment: at least 2 weeks.

Chapter 7: Diets and Their Bad Sides

If you want to lose a few pounds and you want to reduce sugar cravings, then you should not have to go on a diet. As I said, I will guide you through all the dangers they represent. I have experienced negative consequences myself, and I deeply advise you against them.

Magical diets might make miracles, but they certainly do not help with weight loss. Many speedy weight loss methods are only a momentary lifeline that quickly shoots out, and lets us fight with excess weight as we can. Each of us has been on a diet at least once. If you succeeded and lose some weight, it probably returned after the end of the diet. Moreover, there are frequently extra pounds after the failed diet because we need to keep in mind the frustration, and the best way to comfort ourselves is by - eating food!

Eat whatever you want and whenever you want, and watch the pounds disappear! Sound familiar? Although successful diets are a rarity, I will mention five of those which are definite failures.

Diets With Only One Type of Food

For example, a cabbage soup or grapefruit diet - when only one kind of food is consumed for a long time. It is clear how such a diet is harmful, because the body does not get all the necessary nutrients. And after returning to the normal menu, our organism will look for more food to make up for all that it was denied during the diet.

Diets for Cleansing (Detoxification Diets)

Body cleansing products such as a variety of teas and herbal preparations are completely unnecessary and ineffective because our body has its own natural mechanisms – the liver and kidneys that perform the job of detoxification quite effectively, without outside assistance.

Miracle Supplements

Products such as apple juice or green tea and various enzymes, which are said to help the body to burn calories if you consume them after meals, have no effect on weight loss. A product with such a function simply does not exist. It is, of course, just another marketing trick of manufacturers of such products.

Long-Term Fasting and Low-Calorie Diets

Inadequate food intake into the body or too little intake of caloric food has a counterproductive effect on weight loss. Figuratively speaking, the organism, in this case, receives a warning about the food shortages and therefore seeks to preserve part of the food in reserve for a rainy day. But when we return to the usual diet, the body still continues with the storage of reserves for some time, and therefore the pounds accumulate even faster than before the diet.

Also, the pounds lost during such a diet include a loss of fluid, fat, and muscle tissue, while those made after the return of the normal menu consists mainly of fatty tissue.

Dream Diets

A diet that sounds too good to be true (eat anything and still lose weight! Or lose ten pounds in ten days) probably is just that.

The only weight loss secret lies in a simple fact - eat fewer calories than your body burns. This means not only that we need to eat less, but only less caloric food - lots of fruits and vegetables, minimal fat and sugar. If we add the physical activity that burns the most calories, the recipe is simple.

In the event that the need for food is coming from another source - stress, frustration, depression - the solution lies in addressing these problems with them because the false hunger will disappear as well as the need to comfort ourselves with some chocolate.

Dangers of High Protein Diets

As I told you at the beginning, it is this diet that was my choice to get rid of sugar in the body and lose pounds. The chaos in my body left by this diet was indescribable.

In recent years, some of the most popular diets for quick weight loss were the high protein diets with low-carbohydrates.

These diets are characterized by the fact that the largest number of calories is ingested from foods rich in protein such as red meat, fish, eggs, poultry, and cheeses, while foods rich in carbohydrates are avoided or consumed in small amounts.

Although the American Heart Association and the National Association for Education About Cholesterol do not recommend the implementation of these diets, it is still one of the most popular, probably because of the rapid weight loss in the beginning.

How Does It Work?

The goal of most high-protein diets is to cause a state of "positive ketosis" which results in an intense fat burning as an energy source. For this reason, these diets also called the ketogenic diets.

More specifically, the ketogenic diet is a special diet that is based on the state of ketosis, in which the body enters after a certain time during it, by ingesting mainly protein and fat. When the body enters a state of ketosis, the primary source of energy becomes fat instead of sugar.

This occurs when the body gets a certain period of very low amounts of carbohydrates. Once you start the diet, your body goes through several changes. After about 48 hours from the start of the diet, the body starts to use ketones in order to efficiently use the energy stored in fat cells. In other words, the primary energy source for the organism cease to be carbohydrates (i.e., glucose), and their place is replaced by fat, i.e, fatty acids. Because of that, during ketosis, it is not a problem to eat food with higher amounts of fat than it would otherwise seem reasonable.

This kind of diet, however, can have adverse health effects. Many individuals, who eat a diet too rich in animal protein, often have elevated cholesterol, osteoporosis, or high triglycerides.

Chapter 8: The Risks of High Protein Diets

The most common problems and complications associated with high protein diets are:

Kidney Failure

Consuming too much protein is a burden on the kidneys, which can worsen the health status of people who already have kidney problems.

High Cholesterol

There is a known connection between a high protein diet (consisting of eating red meat and dairy products) and high cholesterol.

Osteoporosis and Kidney Stones

A high protein diet promotes an increased excretion of calcium through the urine (more than in those with a balanced diet), which for a long period increases the risk of osteoporosis and kidney stones.

Carcinoma

A high protein diet does not cause cancer, but limits the intake of fruits, vegetables, grains, and therefore the vitamins, minerals, enzymes, fibers, and antioxidants, which are the biggest fighters against various forms of cancer.

Nervous System

The brain uses glucose as a major source of energy. When there is none, there is a change in its function, such as difficulty with performing mental acts and mood changes.

Experts in nutrition and weight loss find that a lot of high protein diets result in more risks than benefits, and that their appeal mainly because of promises of rapid weight loss is not scientifically validated.

In most cases, people would rather choose the crash diet over a definite change in habits and lifestyle. In this way, after losing weight, they may return to old eating habits that cause excessive body weight, which is contrary to the recommendations on healthy weight loss. Weight loss should result in a decrease in the percentage of body fat, as well as to reduce the risk for heart disease, high blood pressure, diabetes, and cancer, not just weight loss for the acquisition of better looks.

Chapter 9: Change of Lifestyle

As you can see, the desire to reduce sugar is not easy. It becomes not only our habit, but we also become physically dependent on it. It disturbs our health and even our overall functioning as individuals in the society.

A Simple and Magical Solution Does Not Exist

Yes, there are foods that are healthy and which can replace sugar, but It takes discipline and a change of lifestyle.

Although I have given general instructions on how to break the addiction to sugar, I'll give you a concrete example, which I am utilizing in my own life. In the morning, after a night when you don't eat, your blood sugar level is the lowest and we should eat a meal that provides a constant increase of sugar to avoid hunger attacks. It is best that this meal contains a combination of protein and complex carbohydrates (bread, pasta) because they are digested slowly.

Some of my personal practice for breakfast is that I eat some scrambled eggs (prepared to your own taste), some fresh vegetables, and two pieces of toast. This is about enough for me to start the day. Fruit also causes relatively rapid rises in blood sugar, and therefore it might be better to eat it in the afternoon after lunch, but with a gap as it is quickly digested and absorbed best on an empty stomach. This will help in the afternoon when our energy is lowered, and will not have such a yo-yo effect on blood sugar as chocolate or ice cream.

The Importance of Breakfast

Most people forget that breakfast is the most important meal of the day, I was among them until recently too. Believe me when I say that I never forgot about lunch, even only to quickly eat something. Basically it is more of an abundant meal to make up for the lack of breakfast, and usually was full of fat and sugar that could help me. As I already said, this meal leads to a rapid decline of satiety and blood sugar, and I would often eat an abundant snack. The fact that I went to the gym was in vain for me.

Although this daily regime diet is wrong, long ago we gained the habits and if you want to reduce the desire for sugar, this is the first thing you have to change.

We neglect breakfast because we are in a hurry to rush to work, to school, to catch a bus, or because we just want to sleep a little longer almost every morning, or finally because we do not want to prepare a meal every morning. No matter what the reason for this behavior, the fact remains that all the food experts recommend changing our consumption habits. We are working hungry, and we rest when we are full. This is our greatest problem.

Breakfast, which most of us don't practice too much, should be fat and caloric. The day should start strong, and we should be fed to handle the physical and mental efforts that await us.

Let us not forget that our breakfast should provide about a quarter of daily needs in energy, building, and protective substances, which are the main components of our food. Most people do just the opposite: Working hungry, resting when full, which is quite wrong. Breakfast should be rich and full of calories, to start the day strong, fed, and that way to satisfy the physical and mental efforts set by our workplace. All other meals, no matter what you are eating are upgrades and additions.

I personally do not avoid meat. I actually extremely enjoy it, but I try to still have a lunch or dinner which will not be a caloric bomb, even when I eat meat This is why I usually combine it with vegetables and spices. In this way, my meals do not only get healthier, but a lot tastier too.

Try avoiding processed meat, such as for example salami, which is full of preservatives. I always try to find fresh meat and fresh vegetables and not to have a monotonous diet.

In essence, treat your body as you treat your mobile phone. In the morning before you leave home, you charge it, to have plenty of power, and then if necessary, you recharge it.

When you combine this developed habit of eating with physical activity and a bit of sports, believe me, you will not reach for sweets or sugar. If you regularly provide your body with everything it needs, you will have no more cravings for sugar or for anything else.

The Secret Is Moderation

What I discovered during my journey and my research is that the secret to healthy living without sugar is actually moderation and balance. It is necessary to examine yourself and to know your needs and how to meet them effectively.

You do not need to exaggerate anything. If you feed your body well, it will send you signals exactly when and what you need. Just listen to your body, and everything will be ok.

Why do I point this out? I emphasize this because I have observed that often we exaggerate healthy things, which eventually leads to the same effect as before.

When you tell someone that a particular food or ingredient is healthy for him, he can often overdo it and eat or drink only that, or some insane amounts of it. This can best be seen in the case of fresh fruit juice.

We all know that fresh fruit juice is healthy, and that we should drink it. But people often exaggerate this. Many people think that fresh juices are good in all quantities and are harmless. However, this is not the case. Same juice can help one person, and also harm the other.

Fresh juices are a bad choice for some diseases. So if you have a peptic ulcer, gastritis and pancreatitis you should not drink the juice of lemons, oranges, apples, currants, or cranberries. They contain many organic compounds, which increase the acidity of the stomach, which can cause discomfort and pain. Consumption of grape juice should be limited if you have diabetes. It contains too much glucose and calories. Remember, many fresh juices also have laxative properties.

After all, they are not healthy for your sugar cravings or for your body if you consume too much. Let's say that you get a full glass of orange juice, for which you have to squeeze around four average oranges. If you eat four oranges, you would likely be full and it will be a little hard for your stomach. Both of those have the same energy value, but you just did not notice this, because you just drank it in two gulps.

You should treat the same way all the sweets that may contain unhealthy sugars. Nobody is saying that you should not eat them at all, but you should know when you have consumed enough, and you need to know to then how to act accordingly.

As I've already said so far, the struggle is for your own health, and therefore happiness begins with a good scare. Fear is one of the biggest motivators.

Conclusion: For The End of Our Journey

The main point and the main advice that I want you to remember is simple:

If you want to get rid of those cravings for sugar and sweets, if you want to make a step towards a healthier life, the first thing you need to do is to get scared.

You must think about your health first, and then your looks. Take my word, healthy people look beautiful.

I speak from my own experience, and from the profound desire to share my experience and knowledge that I have gained with you.

While I was trying to exclude sugar from my diet because of my appearance, I made a lot of bad decisions. I was on a diet that seriously endangered my health. But when I got scared for my health, I started to take the problem about my diet more seriously and how it could affect my health.

That's why I advise you not to look for shortcuts and wonders. Do not submit yourselves to rigorous dieting and fasting. Do not take drugs and chemicals that promise you that you will never want to taste sugar. All that you will gain with speed will leave you with some long-term consequences.

Approach this in the same way as you would approach a building of a house. No matter how nice your house is and how much beautiful and expensive furniture you put into it, if the foundation is lost it will get cracked and it will get ugly. Also, If the roof is leaking, all the furniture that you bought will get ruined. Then you need to reinvest time and money, but the house cannot be repaired to look like it used to before.

The easiest way is to start slowly changing your habits. You have to start to pay attention to the foods you eat. You need to start reading food ingredients a little bit more when you buy groceries at the store.

You must change the way you approach food. Stop eating food on the principle that "it doesn't matter what it is, I'll eat it just not to be hungry". Plan what, when, and how to feed your body.

200 years ago or more, a man might not have to pay attention to these things. Vegetables and fruit were organic, there was no other kind. The land was free from pollution, and air and water were clean. The products had not been treated with so much sugar and chemicals to endure standing on the shelves of stores. Everything was as you take it from nature.

Unfortunately, today this is not the case, so if you want to eat healthy, you need make a bit more effort.

Believe me when I tell you that after a while it becomes a habit.

A plentiful and quality breakfast that will help you start your day will become a standard. A lunch that will help you maintain energy levels throughout the day and a dinner that will not encumber you will become simply a way of life. The road is hard, and it will be tough at first, but trust me it pays out when you go to the doctor, and he is watching in amazement, wondering how it is possible that you are much healthier.

The last advice I have for you is that if you want to get rid of cravings for sugar you have to resort to nature and you have to look at yourself.

Nature has an answer for all your daily needs for sugar, and other necessary ingredients for the healthy functioning of the body.

If you found this book to be useful, then I'd like to ask you for a favor, would you be kind enough to leave a review on Amazon? It'd be greatly appreciated!

Thank you and good luck!

Printed in Great Britain
by Amazon

35653086R00038